ISBN: 978-1-955993-01-2

<u>Table of Contents</u>

Page 1....................Waist basics

Page 2-4....................Eating habits to slim the waist

Page 5-6....................Exercises for slimming the waist

Page 7-9....................Food to avoid or minimize to lose belly fat

Page 10....................Understanding your path to success

Page 11....................Managing cheat meals so you can still make progress

Page 12....................Sleep plan for a smaller waist

Page 13....................How to make waist-friendly sauces/dressings/dips

Page 14....................Planning basic waist-slimming meals/bowls

Page 15....................Belly sabotagers to watch out for

Page 16....................What to buy before cooking waist-friendly meals

Page 17-46....................Belly fat blasting recipes

Page 47....................Appendix (includes Weekly Progress Form, Daily Fitness Goal Tracksheet, and scholarly sources)

Waist Basics

Welcome to your ultimate research-based guide for losing every last inch of your belly fat! Belly fat is no longer a mystery; there's a whole host of studies that found that it has everything to do with our health! Our bodies actually tell us whether we are healthy or not. Just by looking in the mirror and noticing belly fat, we're able to tell that something in our bodies has gone wrong, whether it's inflammation, blood vessel health, hormonal, or metabolic health.

Belly fat is related to our blood vessel and heart health, levels of inflammation in our bodies, and our metabolism involving blood sugar and cholesterol (3)

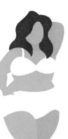

A 33.4 inch waist is considered a hypertriglyceridemic waist in women. That means too many triglycerides! (4)

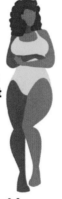

The average waist size is increasing due to a shift in body mass index (BMI) as well as an increase of abdominal obesity.(2,3)

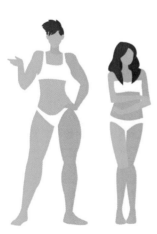

Being skinny doesn't provide much protection either: Even skinny women can have too much abdominal fat if their waists are large and their thighs skinny. Larger thighs and smaller waists have healthier glucose levels. (5) Even if there is no "grab-able" fat around the belly, there can still be fat surrounding your organs! It's all about balance. Also, having larger thighs means you have a combination of more lean tissue (muscles!) and healthy fat.

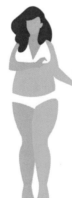

In 2014, the Average woman (who is between 5'3" and 5'4") had a waist size of 38.1 inches (1)

1

Eating Habits for a Healthy Waist

The types of food that we eat actually have specific functions in our bodies. Ultimately, the important thing to remember is that a healthy waist size is easy to attain when your body has all the nutrients it needs to function properly. Without nutrients, a healthy metabolism is impossible. Lots of healthy food items are proven by research to slim the waist. Make sure to include these in your daily diet!

Vegetables reduce risk of heart disease by about 4% per serving (6) - and as heart health improves, the belly fat goes away.

Whole grain consumption is associated with having less visceral (fat around organs) and subcutaneous (grab-able) fat (11).

Green leafy veggies once a day reduce the risk of diabetes (7) - lowering the risk of diabetes can mean less abdominal fat (9).

Carotenoids are waist slimming superfoods that turn white fat into healthy metabolism boosting brown fat - get them from orange vegetables or seaweed! (21)

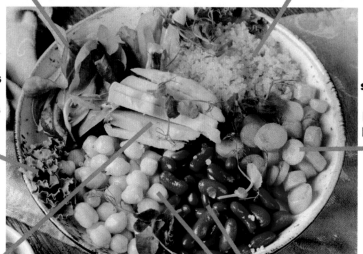

Raw fat like avocado lessens the negative effects of high fat meals on the blood vessels (13,14). Walnuts also have waist slimming and health promoting fats (15). Eat about a handful of raw seeds/nuts per day or 1 avocado a day, it makes a big difference!

Beans significantly contribute to a smaller waist (17) and they get rid of waist-enlarging inflammation. No worries, the bloating is only a phase your body goes through to adjust to the amount of fiber.

Eating Habits:
Handling a Sweet Tooth

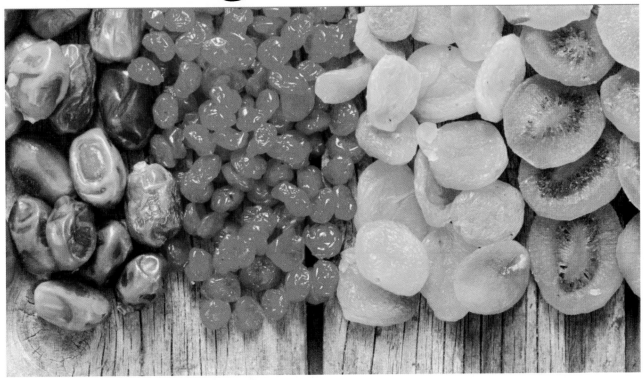

Fruit reduces the risk of heart disease by about 5% per serving (6). Vitamin C rich fruit has also been shown to have waist slimming effects by improving blood vessel health (10).

Dried fruit is waist healthy (12) and sweet enough to replace sugar. Soaking it helps with the texture and it blends well in smoothies and sauces.

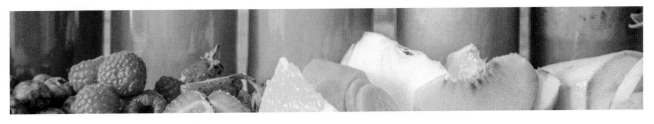

Healthy Doesn't Have to Mean Nasty

Your new waist-slimming lifestyle will upgrade your body, but you don't need it to be a downgrade of a diet. Healthy food can taste really good, just like unhealthy food can! Follow these tips to supercharge your belly fat loss and make health-promoting food that has amazing flavor. Also remember if you still feel like this is too difficult, keep holding on! It only takes weeks for taste buds to adjust and you'll be able to begin to enjoy new flavors (69).

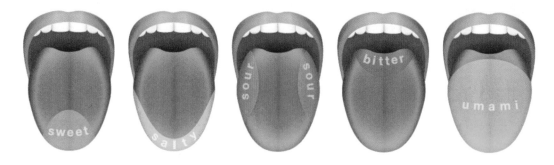

Out of all the ways our tongues are capable of tasting, what really gets us addicted to junk food is UMAMI. But umami is something you can have in healthy food, too. Sources of umami include miso paste (do not get it if it has monosodium glutamate, also known as MSG, in it), mushroom powder, or tomato powder.

Use spices to bring out and add to the flavor, and be okay with using a little salt. When you make your own food, you automatically end up using way less salt than if you bought food from a restaurant or a bag of chips for example.

Certain spices and herbs have belly fat burning abilities. Cayenne pepper is a spice that is known to burn visceral belly fat (19), and it can even extend your lifespan (20)!

Exercise to Target Belly Fat

Some people swear exercise slims their waists while others exercise a lot and still have belly fat. Combining diet and exercise will give you a fool-proof guaranteed way to finally get rid of the belly fat. Here are some research-proven belly fat burning exercises you can do. Choose to do what works for you and make it a regular part of your exercise schedule. Also, the stricter you are with eating healthy, the less exercise you'll need to see a difference.

Along with your exercise plan, it's equally important to maintain muscles so that you continue burning fat (and not muscles). Do this by making sure you're getting adequate veggies and fruit (28), protein (27), and complex carbohydrates (26).

Make sure to do resistance training 2-3 times weekly in combination with aerobic exercise - it's most effective for correcting the body shape or waist/hip ratio (29).

Aerobic exercise gets rid of visceral fat and lowers waist-expanding triglycerides (22).

Visceral fat prevention: 1.8 miles/day
Work off visceral fat: 3 miles/day (23)

What will your exercise plan be?

If you're overweight, you'll likely benefit from continuous aerobic exercise over HIIT, or high intensity interval training (24). This is likely because HIIT may be too high of an intensity for a body carrying around too much weight. HIIT works better for healthy weight individuals as an effective time-saving workout (25).

Exercise to Target Belly Fat

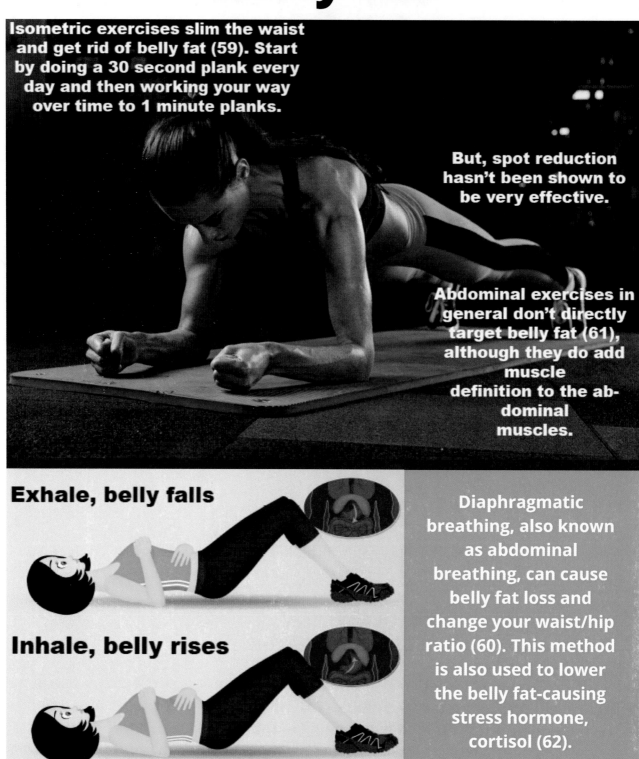

Isometric exercises slim the waist and get rid of belly fat (59). Start by doing a 30 second plank every day and then working your way over time to 1 minute planks.

But, spot reduction hasn't been shown to be very effective.

Abdominal exercises in general don't directly target belly fat (61), although they do add muscle definition to the abdominal muscles.

Exhale, belly falls

Inhale, belly rises

Diaphragmatic breathing, also known as abdominal breathing, can cause belly fat loss and change your waist/hip ratio (60). This method is also used to lower the belly fat-causing stress hormone, cortisol (62).

Food to Avoid
or Minimize

Just like there are certain types of food that help to slim the waist, there are also certain types of food that pack fat around our organs making our waists look blocky... or it can cause fat to pack under the skin creating rolls that we can grab. Some of these types of food add belly fat fast while others can take years before you notice any real gain, and by then you could develop belly-fat related diseases like Type II Diabetes, fatty liver, heart disease, and hormonal issues. Here are the types of food to avoid or at least minimize.

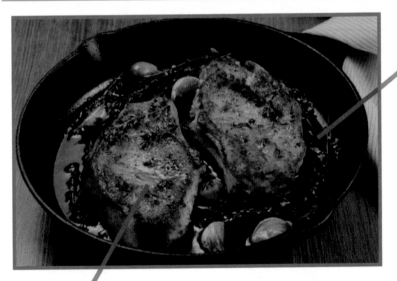

Food that is cooked with oil -even olive oil and coconut oil- (42, 43) impairs blood vessel function.

Healthy blood vessel function is important for a small waist and healthy body weight (58).

Eating meat contributes to belly fat in the long term (47, 48) - this may be due to the presence of POPs that bioaccumulate in animal tissue. POPs are also known as Persistent Organic Pollutants (53).

Alcohol directly contributes to belly fat, and lifetime alcohol consumption adds up. Having moderate consumption at 1 drink per day still results in higher chance of becoming obese (54). Alcohol also makes hips more narrow (55). Beer and spirits contribute to belly fat more than wine (56).

Food to Avoid
or Minimize

It's also important to note that if metabolic issues like Diabetes run in your family, it would be a good idea to avoid drinking your calories in order to maintain healthy glucose levels. If you have a healthy metabolism just make sure it's 100% real fruit juice (64) and no added sugar or high fructose corn syrup.

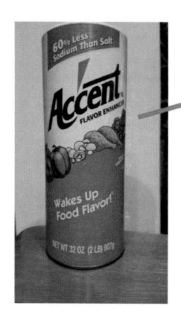

Seems healthy, right? A lot of things that seem healthy, simply aren't. Check the ingredients label for monosodium glutamate or MSG. MSG increases visceral fat (50) and it increases the risk of developing metabolic issues (51).

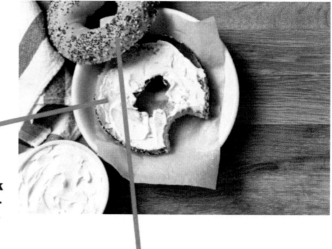

Looks tasty, doesn't it? Is it worth it though? High fat dairy means higher risk of heart failure and increased inflammation, yet appears to be more waist slimming than low fat dairy (45)... still not worth it.

Low fat dairy increases inflammation (44). Consider a bagel with cream cheese to be a cheat meal.

Simple carbs like bread, sugar, crackers, and processed grains like white rice and flour increase belly fat - both visceral and subcutaneous belly fat (57). This is one reason why low carb diets do so well - because they eliminate bad carbs.

Food to Avoid or Minimize

Beware because these ingredients are found in a lot of food items. Salad dressings and barbecue sauce, bread, and other packaged items. Always check the ingredient label!

And remember, when you go out to restaurants to eat, it's likely going to be in that food. So count it as a cheat meal just to be sure.

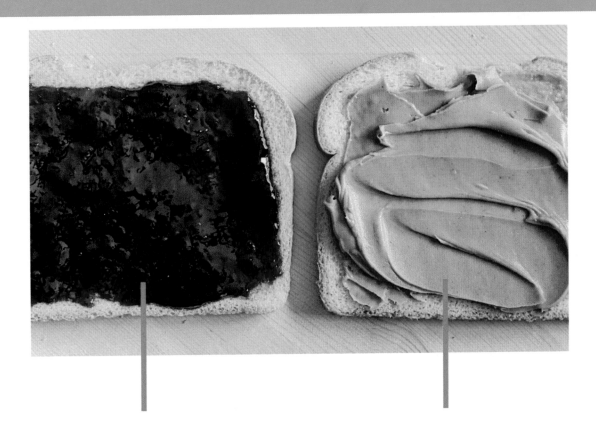

High Fructose Corn Syrup increases lipids and bad cholesterol (52), it also causes hunger (63). So only a couple hours after eating, you'll be hungry again. Sugar also directly contributes to belly fat (53).

Trans fats found in products like peanut butter increase waist size (46). Also be careful with peanut butter because a lot of the time there tends to be oil and sugar added to it. Choose one with just peanuts and salt.

The Path to Success

I can't possibly give you all this information without warning you of what's likely to happen when you begin your waist-slimming journey. There will be sabotage - whether it's your friends, family, or you yourself. Don't take it personally. Remember your goals and come up with a plan for these situations. Failure is not an option. Think of it as more of a journey than a pass/fail challenge. It's time to live your best life! In doing that, we plan NOT to fail. Here are some questions to get you thinking about what you'll do when difficulties arise.

When you get discouraged or tempted, what are some things you can shift your thinking towards in order to improve your mindset (from negative to positive)? What is the current narrative that you tell yourself when trying to make a change? Is it working for you?

What stops you from pursuing health goals (exercising/eating healthy) and what will you do to overcome this in the future?

Remember that failure is normal and is actually a contributing part of success. What is your plan to prevent failure and what is your plan after you've experienced failure?

On your darkest day, what would you say to yourself? What is important to remember during tough times?

What kind of life do you truly want for yourself and how will a healthy lifestyle help you start living that life?

Managing Cheat Meals

So obviously we aren't swearing off unhealthy food for the rest of our lives, but there are some things to consider when planning cheat meals. Cheat meals will make it harder to stick with healthy eating, so a certain level of discipline should be in place when you decide to have your first cheat meal. Here's some information to help you have a plan for managing your cheat meals. It could be ice cream once a month, a burger once every 2 weeks, or a quesadilla once a week. Either way, it should be a frequency that still allows you to see progress from month to month.

Consider the TYPE of cheat meal

- Sugar and simple carbs (processed food)
- Alcohol and soda
- Fatty food (fried food, cheese, oil, etc)
- Processed meat, red meat, poultry

HERE'S A TIP!

Have a fresh avocado with a high fat meal, to help lessen the negative effects (13)!

- What is your favorite type of cheat meal?
- How often will you indulge?
- How might you eat differently during cheat meals to reduce some of the health damage?

After cheat meals, return to your goal-based thinking.

When you go back to a healthy lifestyle, you'll have more awareness of the negative effects of the cheat meals as well as a renewed sense of discipline for reaching your health goals.

No one likes to stay stagnant with their goals, so space your cheat meals far enough apart so that you can see measureable improvements in your waist size over time.

Sleep Plan

Get at least 8 hours of sleep for a healthy waist!

Sleep is super important for a healthy waist size. If you don't get enough, fat will collect onto the belly (39). Make sure to plan your day around sleep and not plan your sleep around your day! The body just needs time to recharge and heal itself. Here's a sleeping plan to make it easier to get that essential waist-slimming sleep.

Don't use alcohol to fall asleep

Alcohol alters your quality of sleep, which results in overeating because of the hormone leptin being increased due to lack of REM sleep (40, 41).

Avoid eating food, drinking beverages, or smoking

No coffee, caffeinated beverages, chocolate, nicotine/tobacco, or sugar. Let your stomach rest, if it doesn't get to rest, it may keep you up at night.

Make your bed and room peaceful

Keep the temperature in your room a little cool (60-70 degrees), make your room dark by covering the light from electronic devices, use white noise like fans to help tune out distracting sounds.

Relax before you go to bed

It's important to get into a mindset that makes it easy to fall asleep. Try deep breathing before you go to sleep. Take a bath, cuddle, or stretch to prepare for bedtime.

Don't exercise right before bedtime

Let there be at least 2 hours between your last workout and bedtime. A workout can really get you going, but you're supposed to be able to go to sleep!

Program yourself

Go to bed around the same time every day. It may take an adjustment period but the body will begin to get its sleep because it is given the right environment to be able to do so.

Most importantly, Be consistent!

Your body will get used to routine, The best thing you can do for your body is give it a chance to adjust to this new lifestyle.

Blending Healthy Dressings/Sauces/Dips

1. **Decide on a Flavor**

Sweet - Add pre-soaked dried fruit

Savory - Add herbs, spices, and salt

Spicy - Add peppers (cayenne, jalapeno, etc)

Vinegary - Add balsalmic or apple cider vinegar

Tart - Add lemon or lime juice

2. **Chooose Nuts/Seeds**

Flaxseeds, walnuts, pecans, etc

3. **Add Vegetables**

i.e. tomato, onion, garlic

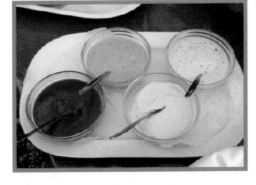

4. **Add Water or Nutmilk**

5. **Optional: Add miso or mushroom seasoning for umami flavor**

6. **Taste and Adjust Flavor with Salt or Seasonings and... Enjoy!**

Planning Basic Meals

Pick from at least 2 categories to create a new meal. Add seasonings, sauce, or dressing, and enjoy!

Mix and Match

Dried Fruit
Raisins
Dates
Cranberries
Goji berries
Yacon syrup
Apricots
Apples
Mango

Fresh Fruit
Cherries
Blueberries
Pineapples
Apples
Oranges
Peaches
Strawberries
Bananas

Raw Fats
Avocado
Pecans
Almonds
Walnuts
Flaxseeds
Pumpkin Seeds
Chia Seeds
Hemp Seeds
Sunflower Seeds

Legumes
Lentils
Peas
Chickpeas
Navy Beans
Kidney Beans
Pinto Beans
Lima Beans
Black Beans
Edamame/Tempeh

Vegetables
Cabbage
Carrots
Onions
Peppers
Kale
Spinach
Brocolli
Cauliflower
Celery
Eggplant

Healthy Carbohydrates
Sweet Potatoes
Quinoa
Oatmeal
Corn
Squash
Whole Wheat Pasta
Brown Rice
Barley
Millet
Yuca

Belly Sabotagers

What to cut back on

Everything listed are major contributors to belly fat. If you avoid all of these things, you can be sure that your belly fat will go away. Of course you'll likely eat/drink these on occasion, but you'll be more aware of the consequences of eating these foods, which will help you to desire them less. Then you can moderate how often you eat these food items.

MSG
Tastes very good but increases deadly visceral belly fat. Found in take-out food, try soy sauce or mushroom seasoning instead.

Fried food
Oil is like sugar, empty calories. Cooked oil destroys blood vessels and leads to health issues.

Most cheese
There isn't much research on cheese, but Gouda appears to reduce belly fat. Otherwise it appears that cheese generally
increases belly fat.

Simple Carbs
Large contributor to belly fat. Simple carbs are missing a lot of fiber and nutrients. Stop eating these and belly fat will melt off.

Alcohol
When drinking, keeping it to one drink and no more is best. Binge drinking causes lots of belly fat. Also alcohol affects sleep, making it more difficult over time to get adequate sleep.

Meat, incl. Poultry
It slowly increases the amount of belly fat over time. Appears to help with weight loss short term.

Caffeine
Affects belly fat in an indirect way: by interrupting sleep. Don't have caffeine after 12 pm in order to get to sleep on time.

Processed food
Sugar, high fructose corn syrup, hydrogenat- ed oils and other weird ingredients that don't sound like real food. One of the largest contributors to belly fat.

Dairy
Increases inflammation, yet appears to decrease waist size when con- sumed whole fat, not low fat. Monitor how often you eat this as it increases inflammation which indirectly causes belly fat.

Flavor Essentials to Buy Before Cooking

1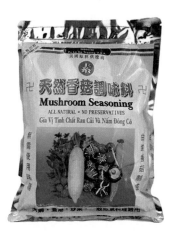

Mushroom Seasoning

2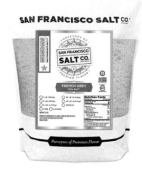

French Grey Salt

3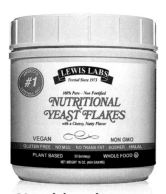

Nutritional Yeast Flakes

4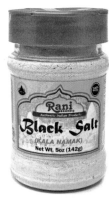

Black Salt

*Can be purchased on Amazon/online

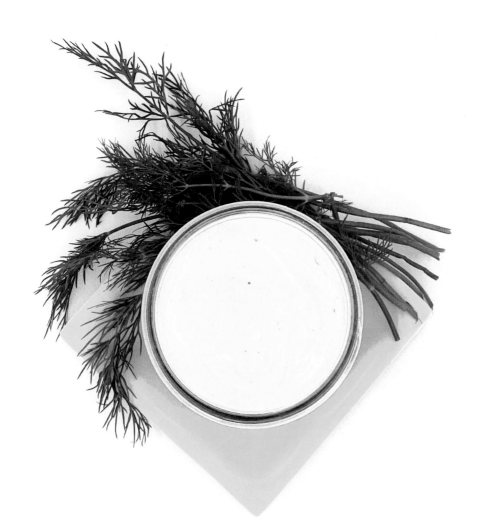

Mayo-Mayo

Ingredients

2 cups raw cashews
1 cup water
juice of 2 lemons
1/2 tsp black salt
1/8-1/4 tsp garlic powder
1/4-1/2 tsp onion powder
1 tsp maple syrup
1 tbsp yeast flakes
1 1/2 tsp french grey salt
1 tsp mushroom seasoning

Directions

Blend and enjoy.

Ranch Dressing

Ingredients

1 cup raw cashews
1 cup water
juice of 2 lemons
2 tsp french grey salt
1 tbsp garlic powder
1 tbsp onion powder
2 tsp yeast flakes
1 tsp dill weed
1/2 tbsp maple syrup
1 tsp mushroom seasoning

Directions

Blend and enjoy on salads, as a dip, as part of a new sauce, etc.

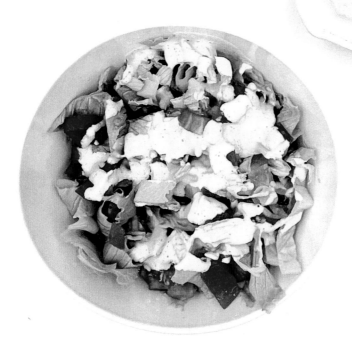

Caesar Dressing

Ingredients

1 recipe Mayo-Mayo (see recipe)
1-2 tbsp capers
1/8 tsp cayenne
1 tbsp kelp powder
1/2 tsp garlic powder
optional

Sweet Potato Onion Soup

Ingredients

2 medium sweet potatoes, peeled and cut into 1 inch rounds
1 heaping tbsp coconut butter
1/2 cup crushed cashews
1 large garlic clove
3 cups water
1 medium yellow onion, chopped coarsely or diced
1 handful of fresh spinach
1 tsp mushroom seasoning
salt to taste

Directions

Blend water, garlic clove, crushed cashews, and coconut butter. Then add all ingredients except spinach into a pot on the stove. Turn heat to medium high until boiling, then cook on low heat until sweet potatoes are tender. Stir occasionally to prevent sticking. Toss in spinach at the end. Salt to taste

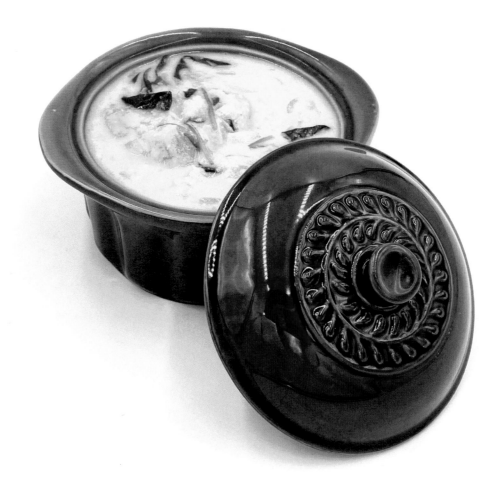

Chickpea Baked Bell Pepper

Ingredients

1 14 oz can garbanzo beans, drained and mashed with fork
1/2 tsp garlic powder
2 heaping tbsp nutritional yeast flakes
1 tbsp mushroom seasoning
2 tbsp diced red onion
2 scallions, sliced
1/2 stalk celery, diced
2 bell peppers with tops cut off and seeds removed (lightly salt inside of peppers)
1/2 tsp salt to taste
2 tbsp rolled oats
1/2 tsp thyme
1/2 cup Mayo-Mayo (see recipe)
Sprinkle of smoked paprika

Directions

Mix all ingredients and fill bell peppers. Sprinkle with smoked paprika. Bake at 375 degrees Fahrenheit for one hour or until peppers are wrinkling and tops are golden brown.

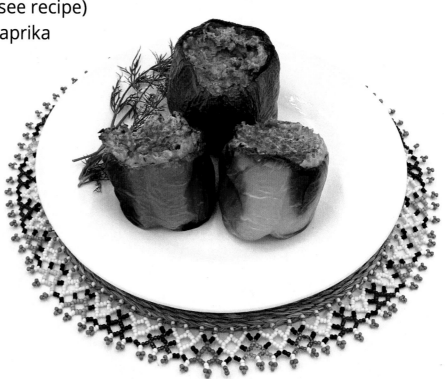

Sweet Pecan Oatmeal

Sauce Ingredients

1 large banana
5 pitted dates
1 1/2 cup water
1/4 cup flaxseed meal

Oatmeal Bowl Ingredients

1/2 cup steel cut oats
1 1/2 cup water
1/2 cup pecans
pinch of salt

Sauce Directions

Blend ingredients.

Oatmeal Bowl Directions

Microwave on high for 3 minutes or boil water on stovetop, stir in oats and then turn on low heat and simmer for about 6 minutes.

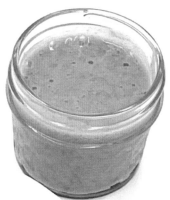

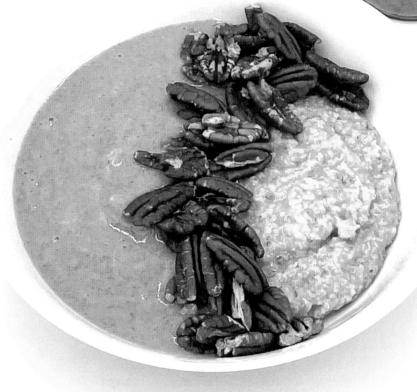

Barley Soup

Ingredients

2 garlic cloves
1 large onion
1 leek
1/2 red bell pepper
1/2 tsp thyme
3/4 cup hulled barley
1 tsp mushroom seasoning
1/4 cup almond meal
generous handful of cut kale
1/2 tsp cayenne to taste
5 cups water or enough to
cover ingredients by one inch
salt to taste

Directions

Cut up garlic, onion, red bell pepper and put in pot. Add seasonings. Rinse barley and add to pot. Add water. Bring to boil, then lower heat. Cover and let simmer. Add water occasionally, if necessary. When barley is tender and chewy, add kale, leek, and almond meal. When kale is tender and still bright green, salt to taste and enjoy.

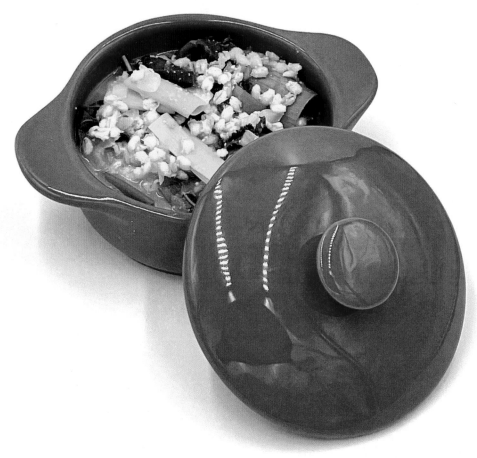

Yellow Lentil Soup

Ingredients

1/2 lb dried yellow lentils
1/2 carrot, diced
1/2 tsp crushed ginger
1 medium onion, diced
2 cloves garlic
1/2 stalk celery, diced
1/2 red bell pepper, diced
1/4 tsp cinnamon
2 tsp cumin
1 tsp mushroom seasoning
water - to cover ingredients, as
needed
1 1/2 tsp salt, or to taste

Directions

Place all ingredients in a pot.
Cover ingredients by about an
inch of water. Boil, then turn the
heat down, and simmer until
ready. Alternatively, you may
place ingredients in a crockpot on
low until the lentils are tender
(should take roughly half a day).

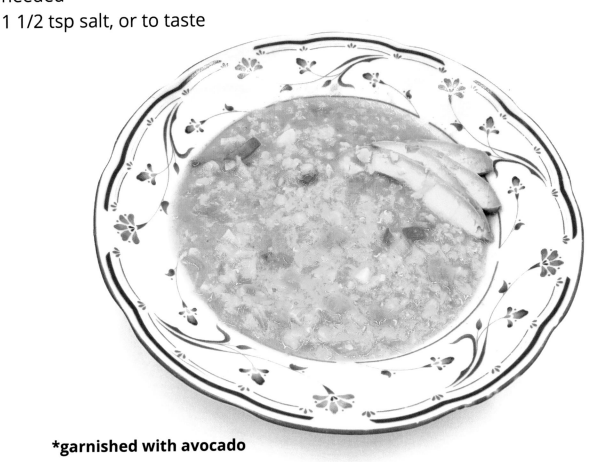

*garnished with avocado

Green Energy Smoothie

Ingredients

3 cups pineapple
2 bananas
1 cup fresh kale
2 cups water
1/4 cup flaxseed meal

Directions

Blend ingredients and enjoy.

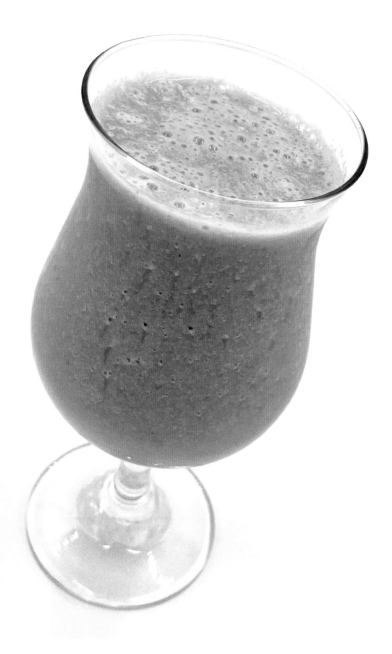

Sweet Heat Sauce

Ingredients

1/3 cup whole flaxseeds
3 1/2 cups water
10 medjool dates
1 tomato
1 tbsp braggs amino acids or soy sauce
1/4-1/2 tsp cayenne pepper
2 fresh lemons, squeeze for fresh juice
1 tsp basil
1 tsp salt or to taste
1 tsp mushroom seasoning
1 tsp garlic powder

Directions

Boil flaxseeds in the water until they develop a thicker sauce-like consistency. Strain the flaxseeds out and then let cool. After cooled, add ingredients to blender and blend.

Whole Grain Pita Sandwich

Fresh Ingredients
1 whole grain pita bread
1 avocado, diced
1 tomato, diced
handful of cut cilantro
1 fresh squeezed lemon
1/2 tsp mushroom seasoning
1/4 tsp salt
Sweet heat sauce (see recipe)

Cooked Ingredients
1 can red beans
1 can black beans
1/2 tsp mushroom seasoning
1/2 tsp onion powder
1/2 tsp garlic powder
pinch of cayenne
1 tsp salt or to taste

Sandwich Directions
Combine fresh ingredients and cooked ingredients, place in pita pocket and add sweet heat sauce and/or mayo-mayo (see recipe).

Cooking Directions
Place cooked ingredients in pot on stove and turn heat to medium. Heat and stir occasionally until beans are ready.

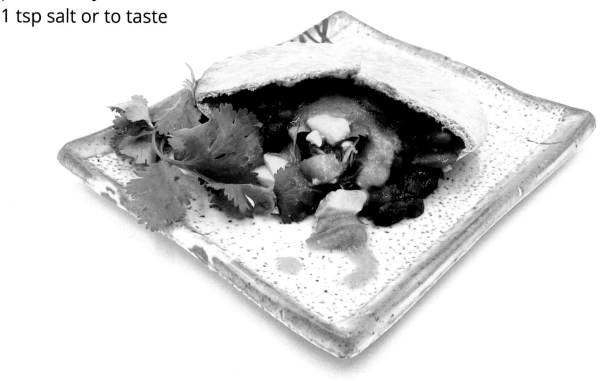

Squash Medley

Ingredients

1/2 avocado, mashed
1 zucchini squash, halved longway
and sliced
1 yellow squash
1/2 medium onion, diced
1/2 orange bell pepper, diced
2 cloves garlic, crushed
1/4 tsp chipotle powder
1/2 tsp smoked paprika (sweet)
1 tsp mushroom seasoning
1 1/2 cup water
French grey salt to taste
Dash of cayenne optional

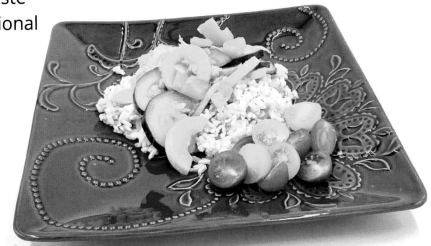

served on a bed of brown rice and garnished with tomatoes

Directions

Mash avocado in pan, place garlic, onion, green pepper in pan on the avocado. Add sliced squashes and top with seasonings. Pour water over veggies. Turn heat on high and cover. Bring to boil, and allow to steam for 5-7 minutes. When finished, serve on a whole grain such as brown rice or whole grain pasta.

Creamy Cilantro Dressing

Ingredients

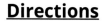

1/4 cup chopped fresh cilantro
1/2 cup water
1/2 cup english walnuts
3 tbsp fresh squeezed lemon juice
3/4 cup crushed pineapple in 100% juice
1 clove garlic
1 tsp salt or to taste

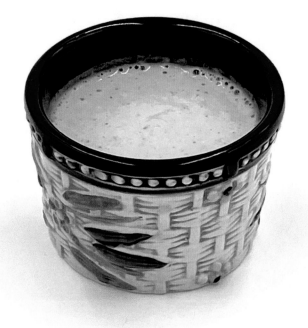

Directions

Blend and enjoy on Buddha bowls, on salads, or as a light and tasty dip.

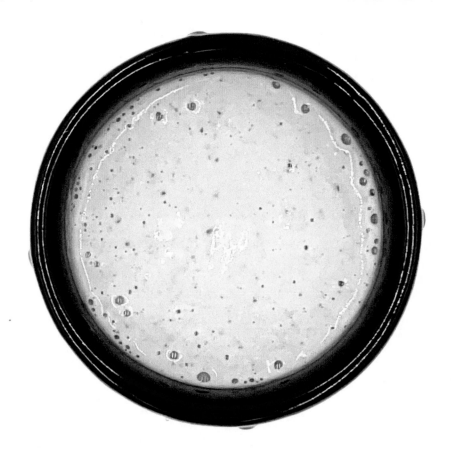

Jalapeno Corn Salsa

Ingredients

2 tsp finely diced jalapeno, no seeds
1 cup diced tomato
1/4 cup diced white onion
1/2 cup sweet corn
2 tsp fresh chopped cilantro
2 tsp fresh squeezed lemon juice
1/4 tsp salt or to taste

Directions

Combine ingredients and enjoy in bowl.

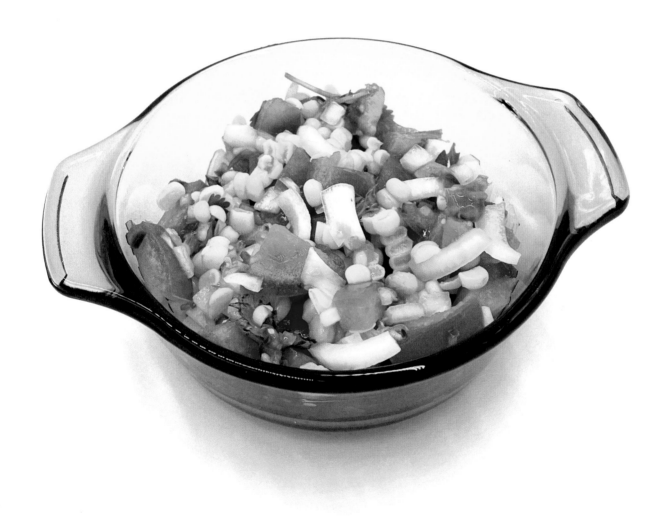

Pink Bean Bowl

Bean Ingredients
1 14 oz can pink beans
1/2 tsp cumin
1/2 tsp salt
1/2 tsp mushroom
seasoning
1/4 tsp chipotle powder
1 clove garlic, minced
1/2 tsp garlic powder
1/2 cup green bell pepper
1/2 cup red onion
1/2 tsp onion powder

Bowl Ingredients
Beans, jalapeno corn salsa (see recipe)
Creamy cilantro sauce (see recipe)
Brown Rice (recipe below)

Directions
Place bean ingredients
in pot on medium heat
and cook until beans are
ready.

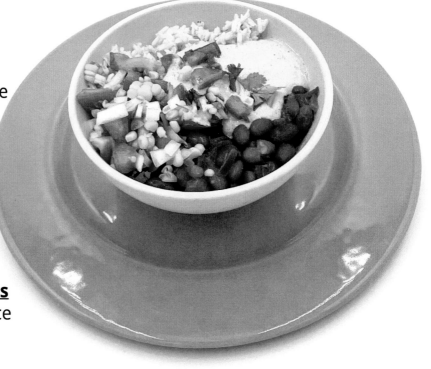

Brown Rice Ingredients
1 cup brown jasmine rice
2 cups water
1/2 tsp salt
1/2 tsp dulse flakes optional

Directions
Place in rice maker or boil and then simmer on low until done.

Pistachio-Lime Dressing

Ingredients

1/2 cup salted pistachios
2 tbsp fresh lime juice
1/2 clove garlic
3/4 cup water
1/4 cup walnuts
1 tsp mushroom seasoning

Directions

Blend and enjoy on salads, and in
Buddha bowls.

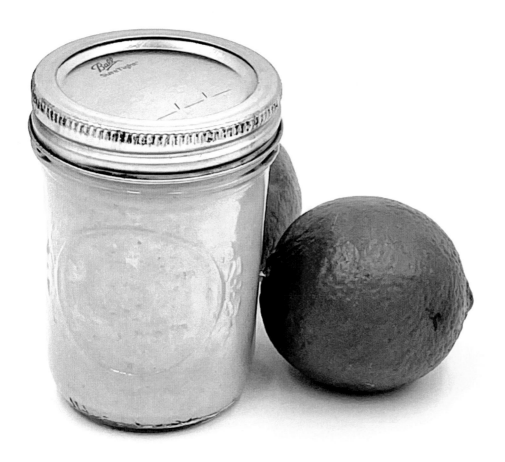

Mango Avocado Black Bean Bowl

Salsa Ingredients
1 avocado, diced
1 mango, diced
1-2 tbsp red onion
1 tbsp chopped cilantro
1/4 tsp salt or to taste

Bean Ingredients
1 14 oz can black beans
1/4 tsp onion powder
1/4 tsp garlic powder
1/2 tsp mushroom seasoning
1/4 tsp salt

Directions
Prepare bean ingredients in pot on stove on medium heat until beans are ready. Mix fresh ingredients together. Serve as a bowl with rice and Pistachio-Lime dressing.

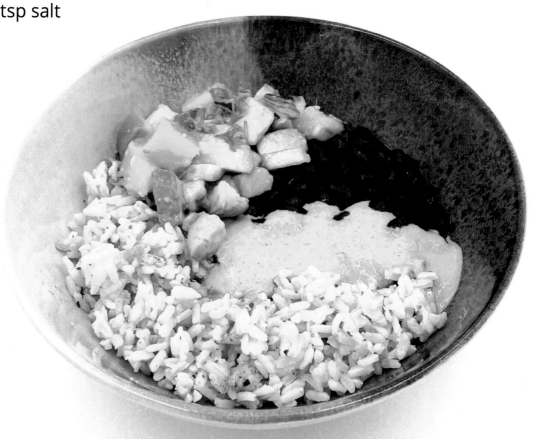

*served with brown rice

Chocolate Craving Smoothie

Ingredients
1 tbsp pure cocoa powder
1/2 tsp vanilla extract
2 large frozen bananas
7 pitted medjool dates
2 cups almond milk
1/4 cup pecans
1/4 cup flaxseed meal

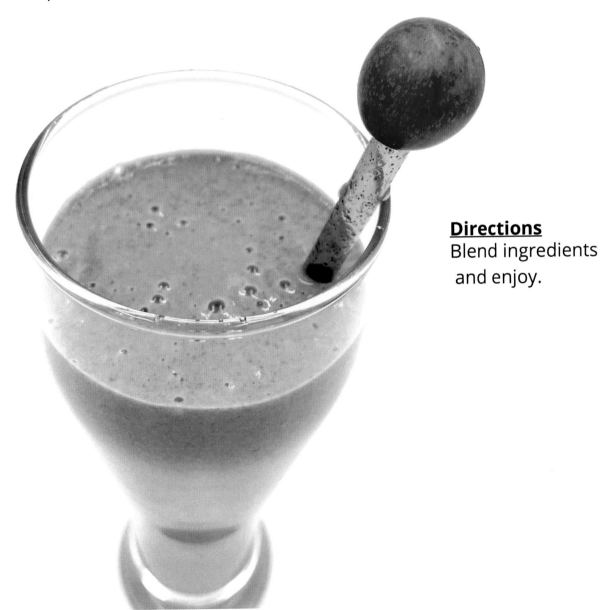

Directions
Blend ingredients
and enjoy.

Veggie Pasta

*Cook 8 oz of dry brown rice pasta according to package instructions. Set aside.

Steamed Veges

1/4 cup diced red onion
1/4 cup red bell pepper
1 cup brocolli
3/-4 black pitted olives, sliced
1 cup water

Steam red onions, red bell pepper, brocolli, and olives on medium/high heat with lid on in water until veggies are tender. Then put on low heat and add sauce.

Sauce

2 cloves fresh garlic
1/4 cup nutritional yeast
1 tsp mushroom seasoning
1/2 cup raw cashews
1/2 tsp onion powder
pinch of cayenne
1 tsp french grey salt or salt to taste
1 1/2 cup water

Blend sauce ingredients until smooth, then place in saucepan with steamed vegetables. Turn heat down to low/medium, and stir constantly until sauce thickens {you may need to add water if it gets too thick). Serve over pasta.

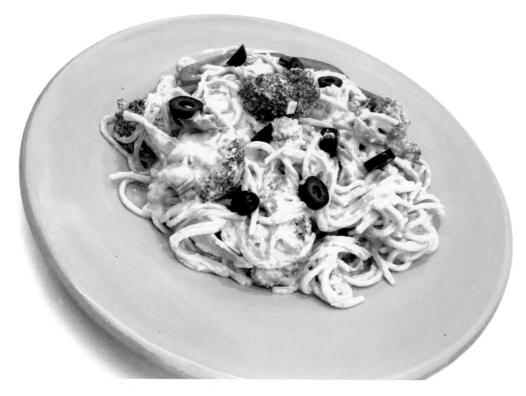

Raspberry Refresher Smoothie

Ingredients

3 bananas
2 cups frozen raspberries
1 tbsp flaxseed meal
3 cups water

Directions

Blend and enjoy.

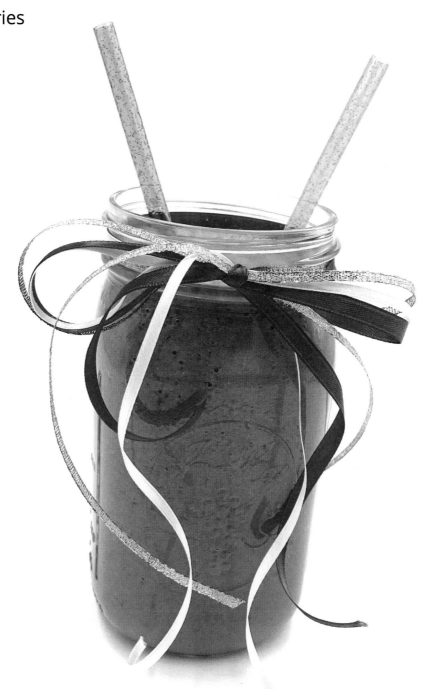

Peaches and Cream Oatmeal

Ingredients

1 cup rolled oats, cooked according to instructions
1/2 can peaches in 100% juice
1/4 cup peach juice
1/2 cup chopped medjool dates
1/2 cup canned coconut milk
pinch of salt
2 tbsp sliced almonds or pecan pieces

Directions

Make oatmeal according to package instructions, adding medjool dates so they can cook together. When oat mixture is done, pour juice from canned peaches into coconut milk and add pinch of salt. Place peaches and nuts on top of the oatmeal mix and pour coconut milk mixture over oatmeal mix. Enjoy!

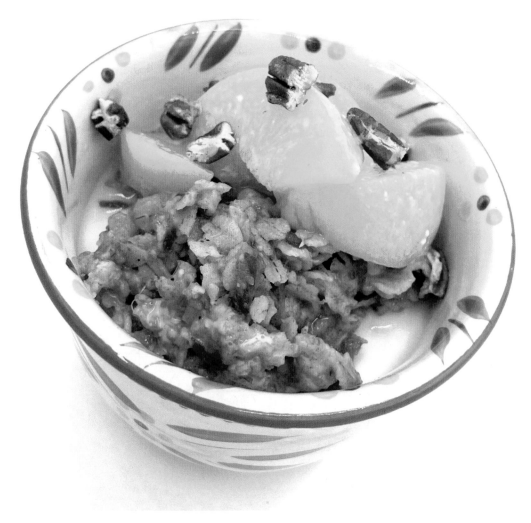

Mushroom Gravy

Ingredients

1 cup sliced white mushrooms
2 tbsp whole wheat flour
1 1/2 cup water
1 tsp onion powder
1 tsp garlic powder
2 pinches of cayenne
1 tsp mushroom seasoning
1 tbsp yeast flakes
1 tsp grey salt

Directions

Place whole wheat flour in dry pan on medium heat, then add water. Whisk until smooth. Add the rest of the ingredients/seasonings. Keep stirring with a wire whisk until the mix thickens.

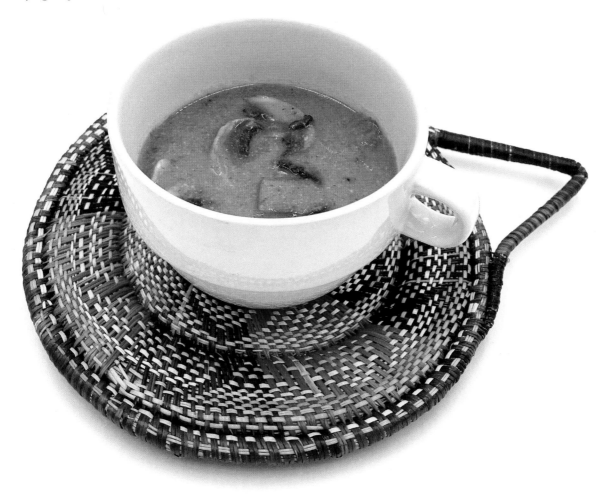

Rice & Peas

Ingredients

1 can of drained pigeon peas
1 can of coconut milk
1 1/2 cups water
1/2 bell pepper, finely chopped
1 medium onion, diced
1/2 tsp celery seed
2 tsp french grey salt
1/2 cup grated carrot
1 tsp mushroom seasoning
1/8 tsp cayenne pepper

Rice

2 cups brown jasmine rice

Directions

Place all ingredients except rice in a pot, and bring to a boil. Add rice, stir, then turn heat to low. Simmer covered for 30 minutes.

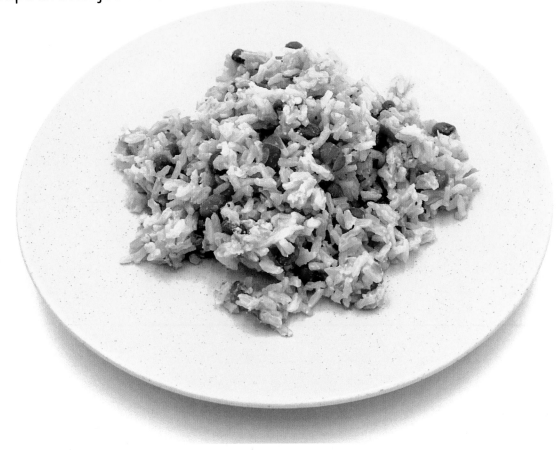

Oatmeal Pecan Patties

Ingredients
2 cups raw rolled oats
1/4 cup pecans, chopped
1 medium onion, finely diced
1/2 red bell pepper, finely diced
2 tsp garlic powder
2 tsp garlic powder
2 tsp onion powder
1/4 cup braggs liquid aminos or soy sauce
1/2 cup nutritional yeast flakes
1 tsp mushroom seasoning
1 heaping tsp sage
1 tsp french grey salt
1/8-1/4 tsp cayenne pepper
1 cup water
1/4 cup canned coconut milk

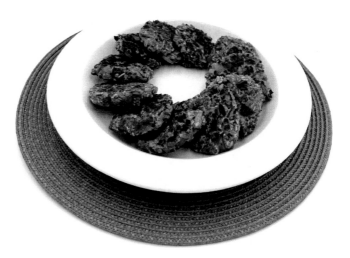

Directions
Place all ingredients in a bowl, adding oatmeal last. Mix well. Let the mixture stand for about 10 minutes until it binds together. Shape into patties and place them on a nonstick pan on medium/high. Cover with lid. Check the patties every 5 minutes to see if they've browned on the bottom, then when golden brown, turn patties over and place lid back on. Continue cooking until other side is golden brown.

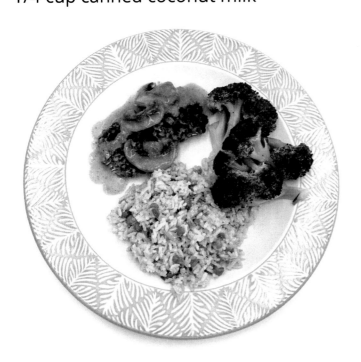

Couscous Stew

Ingredients
2 garlic cloves, minced
1 yellow onion, diced
2 medium yellow potatoes, peeled and cut into 1 inch chunks
1/4 tsp celery seed or 1 stalk celery, diced
1 tsp onion powder
1 can chickpeas
1 tsp french grey salt
1 cup water
1/2 tsp smoked paprika
1 tsp yellow curry
1 tsp mushroom seasoning
1/2 large orange bell pepper, diced
1/8 tsp cayenne
1/2 tsp cumin
1 tsp dried parsley

*garnished with fresh tomatoes and scallions

Directions
Boil ingredients, then stir and turn down to medium/low. Stir occasionally. When chickpeas and potato are tender, dish is ready. Serve over a bed of couscous.

Couscous Ingredients
1 cup whole grain couscous
1/2 coconut cream
1/2 cup water

Couscous Directions
Bring water and coconut cream to boil, then stir in couscous, cover with lid and remove from heat. Let steam for 5 mins.

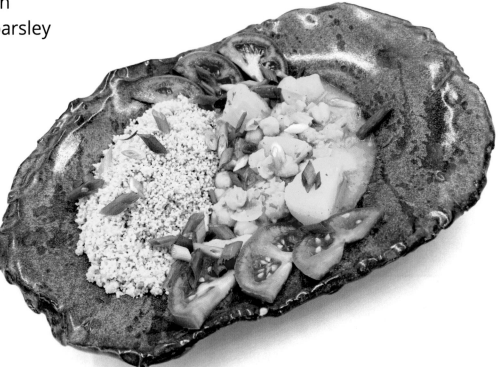

Garlic Sauce

Ingredients
10 medjool dates
2 cups water
4 tsp braggs amino acids or soy sauce
4 garlic cloves
1 tbsp tahini
2 tbsp red pepper flakes
2 tsp mushroom seasoning
salt to taste

Directions
Blend all ingredients except the red pepper flakes. Add red pepper flakes last. Heat, and serve with steamed broccoli (or vegetable of your choice).

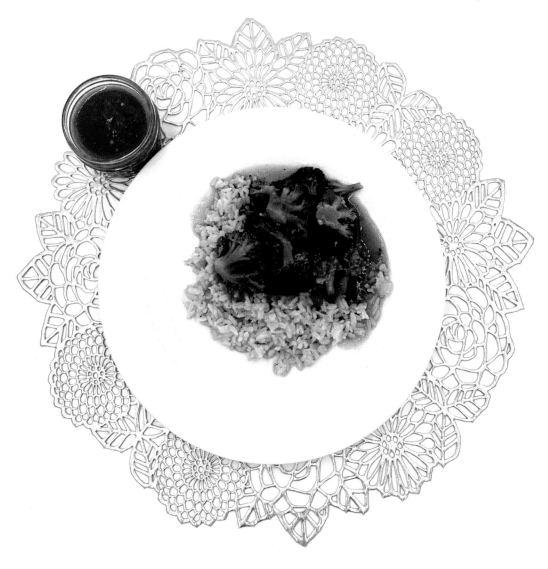

"Cabbards"

Ingredients

1 lb fresh collard greens, thinly sliced
1/2 head cabbage, cut finely
1 large yellow onion, sliced
1/2 dried red pepper, crumbled
1/2 red bell pepper, sliced
3-4 large garlic cloves
2 finely chopped/blended dates in 1/4 cup water
2 heaping tsp mushroom seasoning
1 tsp french grey salt
2-4 cups water

Directions

Place onion, red pepper, bell peppers, and garlic in large lidded pot. Then place collard greens in pot. Add seasonings (mushroom seasoning and french grey salt). Add 2 cups of water and put lid back on. Turn on high heat, bring to boil for 3-4 minutes, then turn greens over and cover. Greens will cook down. Let cook for 5-8 mins again, adding more water if necessary. Then add cabbage on top of mix and boil for 5 minutes. Turn over and cover. Keep covered except to stir occasionally or add water as needed, 1 or 2 cups at a time. Add blended dates to mixture and cook until greens are tender.

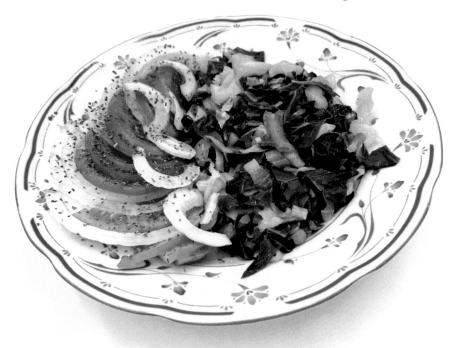

*garnished with white onion, tomato, and basil, can squeeze lemon on greens for different flavor

Lentils

Ingredients

16 oz bag lentils, sorted and rinsed
1 green bell pepper
1 large yellow onion
1 square inch of ginger, crushed and finely chopped
2 heaping tbsp chopped cilantro
3-4 garlic cloves
1 tsp cinnamon
1 tbsp onion powder
1 tbsp garlic powder
2 tbsp cumin
1 tsp chipotle powder
1 tsp smoked paprika
1 tbsp mushroom seasoning
2 large stalks celery
2 tbsp nutritonal yeast flakes
1 1/2 tsp french grey salt
6 cups water
1 tsp salt
1 tomato
2 tbsp coconut butter

Directions

Cover and bring to boil in pot. When it boils, stir, cover, and turn to low. When a lentil mashes easily between your fingers, it's done.

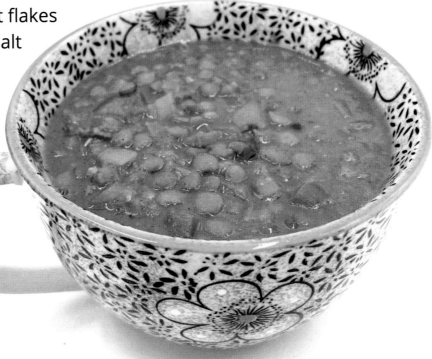

Crockpot Red Beans

Ingredients

16 oz bag red beans
1 large yellow onion, diced
1 green bell pepper, seeds removed and diced
2 large garlic cloves, minced
2 heaping tbsp nutritional yeast flakes
2 tsp mushroom seasoning
1 tsp coconut butter
2 tomatoes

Crockpot Directions

Place ingredients in crockpot on high for half a day.

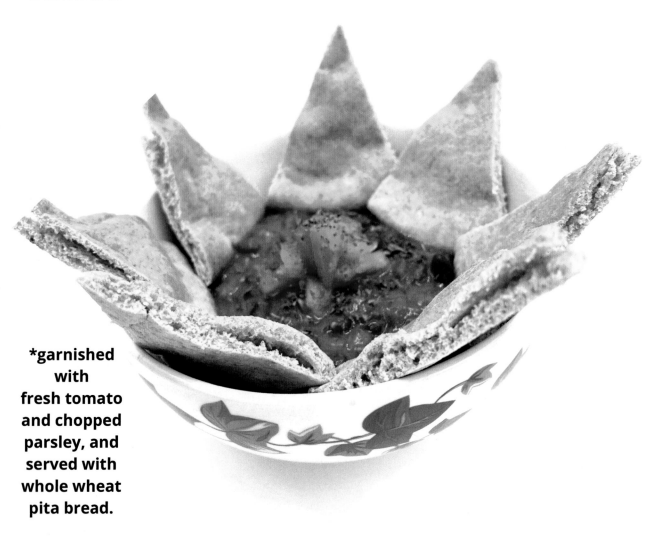

*garnished with fresh tomato and chopped parsley, and served with whole wheat pita bread.

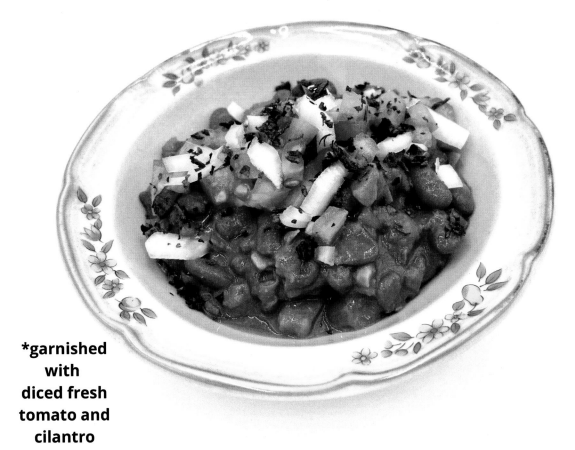

*garnished with diced fresh tomato and cilantro

Chili Beans

Ingredients

16 oz bag kidney beans
3 cloves garlic, minced
2 large yellow onions
2 pitted medjool dates, diced
1 heaping tbsp cumin
1 tsp cumin
1 tsp cayenne
1 tsp onion powder
1 tsp garlic powder
1 can diced pineapple in 100% juice, pour out juice
1 heaping tbsp mushroom seasoning
2 tsp salt
1 tsp french grey salt

Crockpot Directions

Place ingredients in crockpot on high overnight.

Bean Salad

Ingredients

1 bunch cilantro, chopped
1 avocado, diced
1 red onion, diced
1 can kidney beans
1 1/2 cup or about 20-30
cherry tomatoes sliced in half
1 large cucumber, diced
2 cobs of fresh corn, cut off
cob
1 fresh lemon, squeezed
1 tbsp mushroom seasoning
1/2 tsp salt or to taste

Directions

Simply mix all ingredients after prepping them and enjoy.

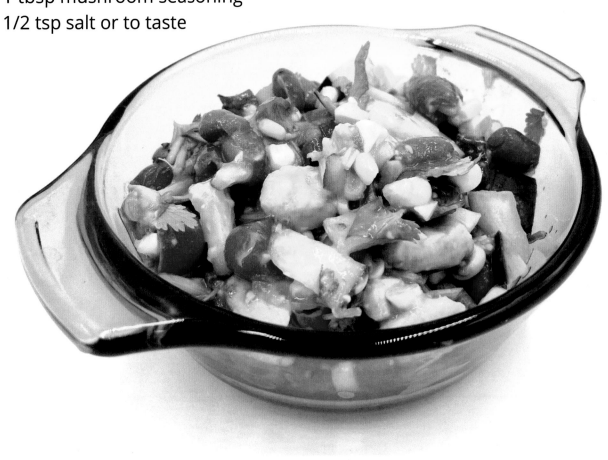

Appendix

Week 1

Waist:_____

Hips:_____

Weight:_____

Body Fat %:_____

Tape progress picture here

*When measuring your waist, make sure it is before you eat breakfast. Stand up straight and place the measuring tape at the smallest point of the waist (near the belly button), take the measurement after exhaling (8). When measuring your hips, measure around the largest part of your buttocks and hips.

What are my challenges this week?

What have I learned or noticed about myself?

How do I feel moving forward into the future?

What are some changes I am ready to make for this upcoming week?

Week 2

Waist:_____

Hips:_____

Weight:_____

Body Fat %:_____

Tape progress picture here

*When measuring your waist, make sure it is before you eat breakfast. Stand up straight and place the measuring tape at the smallest point of the waist (near the belly button), take the measurement after exhaling (8). When measuring your hips, measure around the largest part of your buttocks and hips.

What are my challenges this week?

What have I learned or noticed about myself?

How do I feel moving forward into the future?

What are some changes I am ready to make for this upcoming week?

Week 3

Waist:_____

Hips:_____

Weight:_____

Body Fat %:_____

Tape progress picture here

*When measuring your waist, make sure it is before you eat breakfast. Stand up straight and place the measuring tape at the smallest point of the waist (near the belly button), take the measurement after exhaling (8). When measuring your hips, measure around the largest part of your buttocks and hips.

What are my challenges this week?

What have I learned or noticed about myself?

How do I feel moving forward into the future?

What are some changes I am ready to make for this upcoming week?

Week 4

Waist:_____

Hips:_____

Weight:_____

Body Fat %:_____

Tape progress picture here

*When measuring your waist, make sure it is before you eat breakfast. Stand up straight and place the measuring tape at the smallest point of the waist (near the belly button), take the measurement after exhaling (8). When measuring your hips, measure around the largest part of your buttocks and hips.

What are my challenges this week?

What have I learned or noticed about myself?

How do I feel moving forward into the future?

What are some changes I am ready to make for this upcoming week?

Week 5

Waist:_____

Hips:_____

Weight:_____

Body Fat %:_____

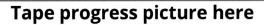

Tape progress picture here

*When measuring your waist, make sure it is before you eat breakfast. Stand up straight and place the measuring tape at the smallest point of the waist (near the belly button), take the measurement after exhaling (8). When measuring your hips, measure around the largest part of your buttocks and hips.

What are my challenges this week?

What have I learned or noticed about myself?

How do I feel moving forward into the future?

What are some changes I am ready to make for this upcoming week?

Week 6

Waist:_____

Hips:_____

Weight:_____

Body Fat %:_____

Tape progress picture here

*When measuring your waist, make sure it is before you eat breakfast. Stand up straight and place the measuring tape at the smallest point of the waist (near the belly button), take the measurement after exhaling (8). When measuring your hips, measure around the largest part of your buttocks and hips.

What are my challenges this week?

What have I learned or noticed about myself?

How do I feel moving forward into the future?

What are some changes I am ready to make for this upcoming week?

Week ___

Waist:_____

Hips:_____

Weight:_____

Body Fat %:_____

Tape progress picture here

*When measuring your waist, make sure it is before you eat breakfast. Stand up straight and place the measuring tape at the smallest point of the waist (near the belly button), take the measurement after exhaling (8). When measuring your hips, measure around the largest part of your buttocks and hips.

What are my challenges this week?

What have I learned or noticed about myself?

How do I feel moving forward into the future?

What are some changes I am ready to make for this upcoming week?

Daily Fitness Goal Tracksheet

	Sunday	Monday	Tuesday	Wednesday	Thursday	Friday	Saturday
Cheat Meal Items							
Sugar or Bad Carbs							
Oils							
Dairy							
Trans fats, MSG, or HFCS							
Alcohol							
Meat							
Caffeine							
Processed Food							
Lifestyle							
# Hours Sleep							
Diaphragmatic Breathing							
# Glasses Water							
Supplements							
Exercise							
Cardio							
Resistance							
Waist Slimming Food Quota							
Seaweed							
Vegetables & Greens							
Fruit							
Healthy Fats							
Healthy Carbs							
Protein							

Daily Fitness Goal Tracksheet

	Sunday	Monday	Tuesday	Wednesday	Thursday	Friday	Saturday
Cheat Meal Items							
Sugar or Bad Carbs							
Oils							
Dairy							
Trans fats, MSG, or HFCS							
Alcohol							
Meat							
Caffeine							
Processed Food							
Lifestyle							
# Hours Sleep							
Diaphragmatic Breathing							
# Glasses Water							
Supplements							
Exercise							
Cardio							
Resistance							
Waist Slimming Food Quota							
Seaweed							
Vegetables & Greens							
Fruit							
Healthy Fats							
Healthy Carbs							
Protein							

Daily Fitness Goal Tracksheet

	Sunday	Monday	Tuesday	Wednesday	Thursday	Friday	Saturday
Cheat Meal Items							
Sugar or Bad Carbs							
Oils							
Dairy							
Trans fats, MSG, or HFCS							
Alcohol							
Meat							
Caffeine							
Processed Food							
Lifestyle							
# Hours Sleep							
Diaphragmatic Breathing							
# Glasses Water							
Supplements							
Exercise							
Cardio							
Resistance							
Waist Slimming Food Quota							
Seaweed							
Vegetables & Greens							
Fruit							
Healthy Fats							
Healthy Carbs							
Protein							

Daily Fitness Goal Tracksheet

	Sunday	Monday	Tuesday	Wednesday	Thursday	Friday	Saturday
Cheat Meal Items							
Sugar or Bad Carbs							
Oils							
Dairy							
Trans fats, MSG, or HFCS							
Alcohol							
Meat							
Caffeine							
Processed Food							
Lifestyle							
# Hours Sleep							
Diaphragmatic Breathing							
# Glasses Water							
Supplements							
Exercise							
Cardio							
Resistance							
Waist Slimming Food Quota							
Seaweed							
Vegetables & Greens							
Fruit							
Healthy Fats							
Healthy Carbs							
Protein							

Daily Fitness Goal Tracksheet

	Sunday	Monday	Tuesday	Wednesday	Thursday	Friday	Saturday
Cheat Meal Items							
Sugar or Bad Carbs							
Oils							
Dairy							
Trans fats, MSG, or HFCS							
Alcohol							
Meat							
Caffeine							
Processed Food							
Lifestyle							
# Hours Sleep							
Diaphragmatic Breathing							
# Glasses Water							
Supplements							
Exercise							
Cardio							
Resistance							
Waist Slimming Food Quota							
Seaweed							
Vegetables & Greens							
Fruit							
Healthy Fats							
Healthy Carbs							
Protein							

Daily Fitness Goal Tracksheet

	Sunday	Monday	Tuesday	Wednesday	Thursday	Friday	Saturday
Cheat Meal Items							
Sugar or Bad Carbs							
Oils							
Dairy							
Trans fats, MSG, or HFCS							
Alcohol							
Meat							
Caffeine							
Processed Food							
Lifestyle							
# Hours Sleep							
Diaphragmatic Breathing							
# Glasses Water							
Supplements							
Exercise							
Cardio							
Resistance							
Waist Slimming Food Quota							
Seaweed							
Vegetables & Greens							
Fruit							
Healthy Fats							
Healthy Carbs							
Protein							

Daily Fitness Goal Tracksheet

	Sunday	Monday	Tuesday	Wednesday	Thursday	Friday	Saturday
Cheat Meal Items							
Sugar or Bad Carbs							
Oils							
Dairy							
Trans fats, MSG, or HFCS							
Alcohol							
Meat							
Caffeine							
Processed Food							
Lifestyle							
# Hours Sleep							
Diaphragmatic Breathing							
# Glasses Water							
Supplements							
Exercise							
Cardio							
Resistance							
Waist Slimming Food Quota							
Seaweed							
Vegetables & Greens							
Fruit							
Healthy Fats							
Healthy Carbs							
Protein							

Sources

1. Fryar CD, Gu Q, Ogden CL, Flegal KM. Anthropometric reference data for children and adults: United States, 2011–2014. National Center for HealthStatistics. Vital Health Stat 3(39). 2016.

2. Fryar CD, Kruszon-Moran D, Gu Q, Ogden CL. Mean body weight, height, waist circumference, and body mass index among adults: United States, 1999–2000 through 2015–2016. National Health Statistics Reports; no 122. Hyattsville, MD: National Center for Health Statistics. 2018

3. Anselmo-Olinto, M. T., Theodoro, H., & Canuto, R. (2017). Epidemiology of Abdominal Obesity. Adiposity - Epidemiology and Treatment Modalities, 1. doi:10.5772/65342

4. Arsenault, B. J., Lemieux, I., Despres, J., Wareham, N. J., Kastelein, J. J., Khaw, K., & Boekholdt, S. M. (2010). The hypertriglyceridemic-waist phenotype and the risk of coronary artery disease: Results from the EPIC-Norfolk Prospective Population Study. Canadian Medical Association Journal, 182(13), 1427-1432. doi:10.1503/cmaj.091276

5. Snijder, M. B., Dekker, J. M., Visser, M., Yudkin, J. S., Stehouwer, C. D., Bouter, L. M., . . . Seidell, J. C. (2003). Larger Thigh and Hip Circumferences Are Associated with Better Glucose Tolerance: The Hoorn Study. Obesity Research, 11(1), 104-111. doi:10.1038/oby.2003.18

6. Fruit and vegetable consumption and mortality from all causes, cardiovascular disease, and cancer: Systematic review and dose-response meta-analysis of prospective cohort studies. (2014). The Bmj, 349(Sep03 18). doi:10.1136/bmj.g5472

7. Intake of Fruit, Vegetables, and Fruit Juices and Risk of Diabetes in WomenLydia A. Bazzano, Tricia Y. Li, Kamudi J. Joshipura, Frank B. Hu. Diabetes Care Jul 2008, 31 (7) 1311-1317; DOI: 10.2337/dc08-0080

8. Waist Circumference and Waist-Hip Ratio Report of a WHO Expert Consultation (Rep.). (2008). Geneva, Switzerland: World Health Organization.

9. Carey, D. G., Jenkins, A. B., Campbell, L. V., Freund, J., & Chisholm, D. J. (1996). Abdominal fat and insulin resistance in normal and overweight women: Direct measurements reveal a strong relationship in subjects at both low and high risk of NIDDM. Diabetes, 45(5), 633-638. doi:10.2337/diabetes.45.5.633

10. García, O., Ronquillo, D., Caamaño, M. D., Camacho, M., Long, K., & Rosado, J. L. (2012). Zinc, vitamin A, and vitamin C status are associated with leptin concentrations and obesity in Mexican women: Results from a cross-sectional study. Nutrition & Metabolism, 9(1), 59. doi:10.1186/1743-7075-9-59

11. McKeown, N. M., Troy, L. M., Jacques, P. F., Hoffmann, U., O'Donnell, C. J., & Fox, C. S. (2010). Whole- and refined-grain intakes are differentially associated with abdominal visceral and subcutaneous adiposity in healthy adults: the Framingham Heart Study. The American journal of clinical nutrition, 92(5), 1165-71.

12. Keast, D. R., Oneil, C. E., & Jones, J. M. (2011). Dried fruit consumption is associated with improved diet quality and reduced obesity in US adults: National Health and Nutrition Examination Survey, 1999-2004. Nutrition Research, 31(6), 460-467. doi:10.1016/j.nutres.2011.05.009

13. Li, Z., Wong, A., Henning, S. M., Zhang, Y., Jones, A., Zerlin, A., . . . Heber, D. (2013). Hass avocado modulates postprandial vascular reactivity and postprandial inflammatory responses to a hamburger meal in healthy volunteers. Food & Function, 4(3), 384-391. doi:10.1039/c2fo30226h

14. Fulgoni, V. L., Dreher, M., & Davenport, A. J. (2013). Avocado consumption is associated with better diet quality and nutrient intake, and lower metabolic syndrome risk in US adults: Results from the National Health and Nutrition Examination Survey (NHANES) 2001–2008. Nutrition Journal, 12(1). doi:10.1186/1475-2891-12-1

15. Song, E., Liu, Y., Kim, H., & Park, H. (2018). Daily Walnut Consumption Favourably Changed Lipid Profiles among Korean Subjects with Higher Waist Circumference. Acta Scientific Nutritional Health, 2(5), 21-25. Retrieved from https://actascientific.com/ASNH/pdf/ASNH-02-0076.pdf.

16. Micallef, M., Munro, I., Phang, M., & Garg, M. (2009). Plasma n-3 polyunsaturated fatty acids are negatively associated with obesity. British Journal of Nutrition, 102(9), 1370-1374. doi:10.1017/S0007114509382173

17. Yanni Papanikolaou & Victor L. Fulgoni III (2008) Bean Consumption Is Associated with Greater Nutrient Intake, Reduced Systolic Blood Pressure, Lower Body Weight, and a Smaller Waist Circumference in Adults: Results from the National Health and Nutrition Examination Survey 1999-2002, Journal of the American College of Nutrition, 27:5, 569-576, DOI: 10.1080/07315724.2008.10719740

18. Hermsdorff, H.H.M., Zulet, M.Á., Abete, I. et al. Eur J Nutr (2011) 50: 61. https://doi.org/10.1007/s00394-010-0115-x

19. Chen, J., Li, L., Li, Y., Liang, X., Sun, Q., Yu, H., . . . Yan, Z. (2015). Activation of TRPV1 channel by dietary capsaicin improves visceral fat remodeling through connexin43-mediated Ca2 Influx. Cardiovascular Diabetology, 14(1), 22. doi:10.1186/s12933-015-0183-6

20. Lv, J., Qi, L., Yu, C., Yang, L., Guo, Y., Chen, Y., . . . Li, L. (2015). Consumption of spicy foods and total and cause specific mortality: Population based cohort study. Bmj. doi:10.1136/bmj.h3942

21. Bonet, M. L., Canas, J. A., Ribot, J., & Palou, A. (2015). Carotenoids and their conversion products in the control of adipocyte function, adiposity and obesity. Archives of Biochemistry and Biophysics, 572, 112-125. doi:10.1016/j.abb.2015.02.022

22. Johnson, N. A., Sachinwalla, T., Walton, D. W., Smith, K., Armstrong, A., Thompson, M. W., & George, J. (2009). Aerobic exercise training reduces hepatic and visceral lipids in obese individuals without weight loss. Hepatology, 50(4), 1105-1112. doi:10.1002/hep.23129

23. Slentz, C. A., Aiken, L. B., Houmard, J. A., Bales, C. W., Johnson, J. L., Tanner, C. J., . . . Kraus, W. E. (2005). Inactivity, exercise, and visceral fat. STRRIDE: A randomized, controlled study of exercise intensity and amount. Journal of Applied Physiology, 99(4), 1613-1618. doi:10.1152/japplphysiol.00124.2005

24. Keating, S. E., Machan, E. A., O'Connor, H. T., Gerofi, J. A., Sainsbury, A., Caterson, I. D., & Johnson, N. A. (2014). Continuous exercise but not high intensity interval training improves fat distribution in overweight adults. Journal of obesity, 2014, 834865.

25. Giannaki CD, Aphamis G, Sakkis P, Hadjicharalambous M. Eight weeks of a combination of high intensity interval training and conventional training reduce visceral adiposity and improve physical fitness: a group-based intervention. J Sports Med Phys Fitness 2016 April;56(4):483-90.

26. Hart, D. W., Wolf, S. E., Zhang, X., Chinkes, D. L., Buffalo, M. C., Matin, S. I., . . . Herndon, D. N. (2001). Efficacy of a high-carbohydrate diet in catabolic illness. Critical Care Medicine, 29(7), 1318-1324. doi:10.1097/00003246-200107000-00004

27. Mettler, S., Mitchell, N., & Tipton, K. D. (2010). Increased Protein Intake Reduces Lean Body Mass Loss during Weight Loss in Athletes. Medicine & Science in Sports & Exercise, 42(2), 326-337. doi:10.1249/mss.0b013e3181b2ef8e

28. Welch, A. A., Macgregor, A. J., Skinner, J., Spector, T. D., Moayyeri, A., & Cassidy, A. (2012). A higher alkaline dietary load is associated with greater indexes of skeletal muscle mass in women. Osteoporosis International, 24(6), 1899-1908. doi:10.1007/s00198-012-2203-7

29. Ho, S. S., Dhaliwal, S. S., Hills, A. P., & Pal, S. (2012). The effect of 12 weeks of aerobic, resistance or combination exercise training on cardiovascular risk factors in the overweight and obese in a randomized trial. BMC Public Health, 12(1). doi:10.1186/1471-2458-12-704

30. The Effect of Vitamin D Supplementation on Metabolic Phenotypes in Thais with Prediabetes. Hataikarn Nimitphong, Rattanapan Samittarucksa, Sunee Saetung, Nuttapimon Bhirommuang, La-Or Chailurkit, Boonsong Ongphiphadhanakul. J Med Assoc Thai. 2015 Dec; 98(12): 1169–1178.

31. Salehpour, A., Hosseinpanah, F., Shidfar, F., Vafa, M., Razaghi, M., Dehghani, S., . . . Gohari, M. (2012). A 12-week double-blind randomized clinical trial of vitamin D3supplementation on body fat mass in healthy overweight and obese women. Nutrition Journal, 11(1). doi:10.1186/1475-2891-11-78

32. Nagatomo, A., Nishida, N., Fukuhara, I., Noro, A., Kozai, Y., Sato, H., & Matsuura, Y. (2015). Daily intake of rosehip extract decreases abdominal visceral fat in preobese subjects: a randomized, double-blind, placebo-controlled clinical trial. Diabetes, metabolic syndrome and obesity : targets and therapy, 8, 147-56. doi:10.2147/DMSO.S78623

33. Teas, J., Baldeon, M. E., Chiriboga, D. E., Davis, J. R., Sarries, A. J., & Braverman, L. E. (2009). Could Dietary Seaweed Reverse the Metabolic Syndrome. Asia Pacific Journal of Clinical Nutrition, 18(2), 145-154. doi:10.6133/apjcn.2009.18.2.01

34. Wan-Loy, C., & Siew-Moi, P. (2016). Marine Algae as a Potential Source for Anti-Obesity Agents. Marine drugs, 14(12), 222. doi:10.3390/md14120222

35. Meissner, H. O., Kedzia, B., Mrozikiewicz, P. M., & Mscisz, A. (2006). Short and long-term physiological responses of male and female rats to two dietary levels of pre-gelatinized maca (lepidium peruvianum chacon). International journal of biomedical science : IJBS, 2(1), 13-28.

36. Kazazis, C. E., Evangelopoulos, A. A., Kollas, A., & Vallianou, N. G. (2014). The therapeutic potential of milk thistle in diabetes. The review of diabetic studies : RDS, 11(2), 167-74.

37. Lehtonen, H., Suomela, J., Tahvonen, R., Yang, B., Venojärvi, M., Viikari, J., & Kallio, H. (2011). Different berries and berry fractions have various but slightly positive effects on the associated variables of metabolic diseases on overweight and obese women. European Journal of Clinical Nutrition, 65(3), 394-401. doi:10.1038/ejcn.2010.268

38. Wang, H., Wen, Y., Du, Y., Yan, X., Guo, H., Rycroft, J. A., . . . Mela, D. J. (2009). Effects of Catechin Enriched Green Tea on Body Composition. Obesity, 18(4), 773-779. doi:10.1038/oby.2009.256

39. Theorell-Haglöw, J., Berne, C., Janson, C., Sahlin, C., & Lindberg, E. (2010). Associations between Short Sleep Duration and Central Obesity in Women. Sleep, 33(5), 601-610. doi:10.1093/sleep/33.5.593

40. Ebrahim, I. O., Shapiro, C. M., Williams, A. J., & Fenwick, P. B. (2013). Alcohol and Sleep I: Effects on Normal Sleep. Alcoholism: Clinical and Experimental Research, 37(4). doi:10.1111/acer.12006

41. Beccuti, G., & Pannain, S. (2011). Sleep and obesity. Current opinion in clinical nutrition and metabolic care, 14(4), 402-12.

42. Rueda-Clausen, C. F., Silva, F. A., Lindarte, M. A., Villa-Roel, C., Gomez, E., Gutierrez, R., . . . López-Jaramillo, P. (2007). Olive, soybean and palm oils intake have a similar acute detrimental effect over the endothelial function in healthy young subjects. Nutrition, Metabolism and Cardiovascular Diseases, 17(1), 50-57. doi:10.1016/j.numecd.2005.08.008

43. Hamsi, M. A., Othman, F., Das, S., Kamisah, Y., Thent, Z. C., Qodriyah, H. M., . . . Jaarin, K. (2015). Effect of consumption of fresh and heated virgin coconut oil on the blood pressure and inflammatory biomarkers: An experimental study in Sprague Dawley rats. Alexandria Journal of Medicine, 51(1), 53-63. doi:10.1016/j.ajme.2014.02.002

44. Meijl, L. E., & Mensink, R. P. (2010). Effects of low-fat dairy consumption on markers of low-grade systemic inflammation and endothelial function in overweight and obese subjects: An

intervention study. British Journal of Nutrition, 104(10), 1523-1527. doi:10.1017/s0007114510002515

45. Nettleton, J. A., Steffen, L. M., Loehr, L. R., Rosamond, W. D., & Folsom, A. R. (2008). Incident Heart Failure Is Associated with Lower Whole-Grain Intake and Greater High-Fat Dairy and Egg Intake in the Atherosclerosis Risk in Communities (ARIC) Study. Journal of the American Dietetic Association, 108(11), 1881-1887. doi:10.1016/j.jada.2008.08.015

46. Pauline Koh-Banerjee, Nain-Feng Chu, Donna Spiegelman, Bernard Rosner, Graham Colditz, Walter Willett, Eric Rimm; Prospective study of the association of changes in dietary intake, physical activity, alcohol consumption, and smoking with 9-y gain in waist circumference among 16 587 US men, The American Journal of Clinical Nutrition, Volume 78, Issue 4, 1 October 2003, Pages 719–727, https://doi.org/10.1093/ajcn/78.4.719

47. Wang, Y., & Beydoun, M. A. (2009). Meat consumption is associated with obesity and central obesity among US adults. International Journal of Obesity, 33(6), 621-628. doi:10.1038/ijo.2009.45

48. Wang, Y., & Beydoun, M. A. (2009). Meat consumption is associated with obesity and central obesity among US adults. International Journal of Obesity, 33(6), 621-628. doi:10.1038/ijo.2009.45

49. Persistent organic pollutants (POPs). (2014, June 20). Retrieved from https://www.who.int/foodsafety/areas_work/chemical-risks/pops/en/

50. He, K., Zhao, L., Daviglus, M. L., Dyer, A. R., Horn, L. V., Garside, D., . . . Stamler, J. (2008). Association of Monosodium Glutamate Intake With Overweight in Chinese Adults: The INTERMAP Study. Obesity, 16(8), 1875-1880. doi:10.1038/oby.2008.274

51. Insawang, T., Selmi, C., Cha'On, U., Pethlert, S., Yongvanit, P., Areejitranusorn, P., . . . Hammock, B. D. (2012). Monosodium glutamate (MSG) intake is associated with the prevalence of metabolic syndrome in a rural Thai population. Nutrition & Metabolism, 9(1), 50. doi:10.1186/1743-7075-9-50

52. Kimber L Stanhope, Valentina Medici, Andrew A Bremer, Vivien Lee, Hazel D Lam, Marinelle V Nunez, Guoxia X Chen, Nancy L Keim, Peter J Havel; A dose-response study of consuming high-fructose corn syrup–sweetened beverages on lipid/lipoprotein risk factors for cardiovascular disease in young adults, The American Journal of Clinical Nutrition, Volume 101, Issue 6, 1 June 2015, Pages 1144–1154, https://doi.org/10.3945/ajcn.114.100461

53. Maria Maersk, Anita Belza, Hans Stødkilde-Jørgensen, Steffen Ringgaard, Elizaveta Chabanova, Henrik Thomsen, Steen B Pedersen, Arne Astrup, Bjørn Richelsen; Sucrose-sweetened beverages increase fat storage in the liver, muscle, and visceral fat depot: a 6-mo randomized intervention study, The American Journal of Clinical Nutrition, Volume 95, Issue 2, 1 February 2012, Pages 283–289, https://doi.org/10.3945/ajcn.111.022533

54. Lourenço, S., Oliveira, A., & Lopes, C. (2012). The effect of current and lifetime alcohol consumption on overall and central obesity. European Journal of Clinical Nutrition, 66(7), 813-818. doi:10.1038/ejcn.2012.20

55. Tolstrup, J. S., Heitmann, B. L., Tjønneland, A. M., Overvad, O. K., Sørensen, T. I., & Grønbæk, M. N. (2005). The relation between drinking pattern and body mass index and waist and hip circumference. International Journal of Obesity, 29(5), 490-497. doi:10.1038/sj.ijo.0802874

56. Halkjær, J., Sørensen, T., Tjønneland, A., Togo, P., Holst, C., & Heitmann, B. (2004). Food and drinking patterns as predictors of 6-year BMI-adjusted changes in waist circumference. British Journal of Nutrition, 92(4), 735-748. doi:10.1079/BJN20041246

57. McKeown, N. M., Troy, L. M., Jacques, P. F., Hoffmann, U., O'Donnell, C. J., & Fox, C. S. (2010). Whole- and refined-grain intakes are differentially associated with abdominal visceral

and subcutaneous adiposity in healthy adults: the Framingham Heart Study. The American journal of clinical nutrition, 92(5), 1165-71.

58. Brook, R. D., Bard, R. L., Rubenfire, M., Ridker, P. M., & Rajagopalan, S. (2001). Usefulness of visceral obesity (waist/hip ratio) in predicting vascular endothelial function in healthy overweight adults. The American Journal of Cardiology, 88(11), 1264-1269. doi:10.1016/s0002-9149(01)02088-4

59. Mohr, D. R. (1965). Changes in Waistline and Abdominal Girth and Subcutaneous Fat following Isometric Exercises. Research Quarterly. American Association for Health, Physical Education and Recreation, 36(2), 168-173. doi:10.1080/10671188.1965.10614676

60. Kwak, Y., & Kim, Y. (2010). The Effect of Abdominal Breathing Exercise on Weight and Body Fat, BMI, Waist Hip Ratio in Obese College Student. Journal of Life Science, 20(12), 1867-1871. doi:10.5352/jls.2010.20.12.1867

61. Kordi, R., Dehghani, S., Noormohammadpour, P., Rostami, M., & Mansournia, M. A. (2015). Effect of Abdominal Resistance Exercise on Abdominal Subcutaneous Fat of Obese Women: A Randomized Controlled Trial Using Ultrasound Imaging Assessments. Journal of Manipulative and Physiological Therapeutics, 38(3), 203-209. doi:10.1016/j.jmpt.2014.12.004

62. Ma, X., Yue, Z., Gong, Z., Zhang, H., Duan, N., Shi, Y., . . . Li, Y. (2017). The Effect of Diaphragmatic Breathing on Attention, Negative Affect and Stress in Healthy Adults. Frontiers in Psychology, 8. doi:10.3389/fpsyg.2017.00874

63. Lowette, K., Roosen, L., Tack, J., & Berghe, P. V. (2015). Effects of High-Fructose Diets on Central Appetite Signaling and Cognitive Function. Frontiers in Nutrition, 2. doi:10.3389/fnut.2015.00005

64. Pereira, M. A., & Fulgoni, V. L. (2010). Consumption of 100% Fruit Juice and Risk of Obesity and Metabolic Syndrome: Findings from the National Health and Nutrition Examination Survey 1999–2004. Journal of the American College of Nutrition, 29(6), 625-629. doi:10.1080/07315724.2010.10719901

65. Abutair, A. S., Naser, I. A., & Hamed, A. T. (2016). Soluble fibers from psyllium improve glycemic response and body weight among diabetes type 2 patients (randomized control trial). Nutrition Journal, 15(1). doi:10.1186/s12937-016-0207-4

66. Abutair, A. S., Naser, I. A., & Hamed, A. T. (2018). The Effect of Soluble Fiber Supplementation on Metabolic Syndrome Profile among Newly Diagnosed Type 2 Diabetes Patients. Clinical Nutrition Research, 7(1), 31. doi:10.7762/cnr.2018.7.1.31

67. Genta, S., Cabrera, W., Habib, N., Pons, J., Carillo, I. M., Grau, A., & Sánchez, S. (2009). Yacon syrup: Beneficial effects on obesity and insulin resistance in humans. Clinical Nutrition, 28(2), 182-187. doi:10.1016/j.clnu.2009.01.013

68. Lehtonen, H., Suomela, J., Tahvonen, R., Yang, B., Venojärvi, M., Viikari, J., & Kallio, H. (2011). Different berries and berry fractions have various but slightly positive effects on the associated variables of metabolic diseases on overweight and obese women. European Journal of Clinical Nutrition, 65(3), 394-401. doi:10.1038/ejcn.2010.268

69. Grieve, F. G., & Weg, M. W. (2003). Desire to Eat High-and Low-Fat Foods Following a Low-Fat Dietary Intervention. Journal of Nutrition Education and Behavior, 35(2), 98-104. doi:10.1016/s1499-4046(06)60046-8

Made in the USA
Monee, IL
16 September 2022

14075744R00043